Sleep Mastery

Practical Solutions For Better Sleep

By Michele Gilbert

<u>Visit My Amazon Author Page</u>

Dedicated to those who choose to stretch beyond their own limits
and to seek a more abundant and fulfilling life.

Your thoughts are creative.

Michele Gilbert

My Free Gift To You!

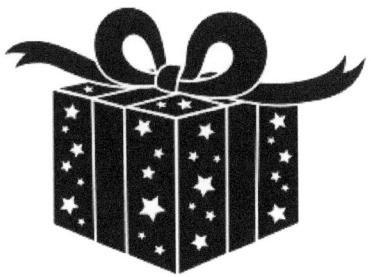

As a way of saying thank you for downloading my book, I am willing to give you access to a selected group of readers who (every week or so) receive inspiring, life-changing kindle books at deep discounts, and sometimes even absolutely free.

Wouldn't it be great to get amazing Kindle offers delivered directly to your inbox?

Wouldn't it be great to be the first to know when I'm releasing new fresh and above all sharply discounted content?

But why would I so something like this?

Why would I offer my books at such a low price and even give them away for free when they took me countless hours to produce?

Simple.... because I want to spread the word!

For a few short days Amazon allows Kindle authors to promote their newly released books by offering them deeply discounted (up to 70% price discounts and even for free. This allows us to spread the word extremely quickly allowing users to download thousands and thousands of copies in a very short period of time.

Once the timeframe has passed, these books will revert back to their normal selling price. That's why you will benefit from being the first to know when they can be downloaded for free!

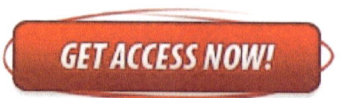

So are you ready to claim your weekly Kindle books?

You are just one click away! Follow the link below and sign up to start receiving awesome content

Thank you and Enjoy!

Tables of contents

Introduction

Thank you so much for downloading my book, "Sleep Mastery" Practical Solutions To Better Sleep"

I know, the title may seem a little brazen, who can really master sleep? But can't any habit be mastered and don't they call it the sleep habit?

If you are not getting enough sleep or not sleeping well .That is not OK. Honestly, there is a big price to pay. I am sure you know that chronic lack of sleep for whatever reason, affects your health, career success, your safety, and yes even your relationships and sex life.

There are many causes for your inability to sleep. It could be just as simple as daily stresses, or we substitute sleep for more work or more play. Some may have medical or mental health conditions that wreak havoc with our sleep

I have tried to show, in very easy ways, some steps and strategies that can change your sleeping rhythm in order to live a restful life. And make everyone else around you happy.

I have tried to explain causes and types of sleeping disorders backed by scientific research and show different approaches in treating some problems. I have offered some techniques, if used with some regularity can change your sleeping habits, plus there are other alternative methods such as diet, yoga, acupuncture, different types of massages and exercises that you can try out anywhere anytime.

Ok...First The Definition...What Is Insomnia?

Do you struggle to sleep no matter how tired you are? Are you anxious when you have to get to bed but you fear you will not be able to sleep? Do you wake up in the middle of the night and stare at the clock knowing you will have to get up for work, but still cannot get any rest? If the answer to this question is yes, then you suffer from the sleeping disorder commonly known as insomnia. This problem is very common and can be caused by many different reasons and factors. The problem is that the condition leads to a constant chronic tiredness and prevents you in your everyday activities because it takes a toll on your mood, energy and even proper functioning of your body. If this becomes a chronic condition you are at risk of developing serious health related problems. It is proven that simple changes to your daily routine and habits can help you overcome this sleep problem. Sleeping pills and medication often lead to addiction that can be even more serious than your initial problem. That is why I prefer to offer a more natural holistic way to treat this condition.

Insomnia is defined as the inability to get enough rest during the night in order to feel rested after waking up. Because everyone is unique and needs different amounts of sleep there is not a strict definition of this condition. Insomnia is more about the relation between the quality of your sleep and the way you feel after waking up, not to the amount of hours you sleep. Even if you sleep enough for every medical standard, 8 hours, if you do not feel rested and still have a feeling of drowsiness and fatigue after waking up it is possible that you suffer from this condition. Insomnia is not a disease; it is a symptom that directs to other disorders, which can be developed by different causes. A sleeping disorder can have simple causes as drinking too much caffeine during the day, but also some serious medical problems of physical or psychological nature.

Symptoms of insomnia:

- difficulty falling asleep, even though you are tired
- frequent waking up during the night
- inability to fall asleep after you woke up
- exhausting sleep

- relying on chemical substances, such as alcohol, cannabis or sleeping pills, in order to get a sound sleep
- waking up too early in the morning even though you do not have too
- daytime drowsiness, fatigue or tiredness
- inability to fully concentrate on your day-to-day tasks

Insomnia can be separated into three types:

Transient insomnia - when symptoms can last from a few days to a couple of weeks.

Acute insomnia – can also be called short-term insomnia. Symptoms can persist for several weeks.

Chronic insomnia - this type can last for months, and sometimes years. Most chronic insomnia cases are secondary, that means they are side effects or symptoms of some other problem.

Insomnia can affect people at any age, but interestingly, it is more common in adult females than adult males. Not sure why but that's what The National Institute of Health studies show. They have also shown it can lead to obesity, anxiety and depression irritability, concentration problems, memory problems, poor immune system function, and reduced reaction time

So that's a pretty good definition of not sleeping well. Do you see how important it is to the quality of your life?

It wasn't until Arianna Huffington fell and hit her face on her desk and almost blead to death that she realized she was working way too much and sleeping way too little. If you are able try to check out her book "Thrive" or watch her Ted Talk on You Tube. Brilliant!

Yes... But What Causes Insomnia?

As with any other medical condition in order to address and treat the problem you should figure out what is causing it. Still, you should know that most sleeping disorders are caused by stress, anxiety and depression. But, on the other hand, your daytime habits and physical health can play a crucial role. There are some questions that you should try to answer in order to figure out what is leading you to this condition.

- Are you under a lot of stress and pressure?
- Are you depressed, or do you feel emotionally blank or flat?
- Do you struggle with constant anxiety and worries when you are awake?
- Have you gone through a traumatic experience?
- Are you taking any medications? There are some drugs that can cause sleep problems as a side effect.
- Do you have any health problems?
- Is your sleep environment quiet and does it suits your needs?
- Do you spend enough time on natural sunlight during the day?
- Have you tried to figure out what is your natural biological rhythm in order to fall asleep and wake up every day in approximately the same time?

Sometimes sleeping problems only last for couple of days and then disappear. This happens when insomnia is tied to a current problem, when the problem is solved insomnia stops. But, if you experience troubles sleeping for a longer period of time, then you suffer from a chronic condition that can be caused by:

- **Psychological issues:** most commonly depression, anxiety, bipolar disorder, post-traumatic syndrome. In order to get rid of your sleeping disorder you should get rid of the cause, and in this case you should seek for professional help of a therapist.
- **Medications that can cause insomnia:** antidepressants, cold and flu medications that contain alcohol, pain relievers that contain caffeine, diuretics, high blood pressure medications.
- **Medical problems that can cause insomnia:** asthma, allergies, Parkinson`s disease, kidney disease, cancer, chronic pain. In this case you should address your physical problem.

- Sleep disorder that can cause insomnia: sleep apnea, narcolepsy, restless legs syndrome.

Who is more likely to suffer from insomnia than others?

Travelers
Shift workers with frequent changes in shifts
The elderly
Drug users
Adolescent or young adult students
Pregnant women
Menopausal women
People with mental health disorders

The Secret Sauce To Improve Your Sleep

In coping with insomnia people tend to unconsciously make their condition worse by taking actions that they believe would help. One might be using sleeping pills. In the long term that could actually worsen the problem.

Often, only a few corrections to your behavior and habits can help you overcome the condition and stop insomnia. A few days of your new routine would have to pass before you notice the changes in your rhythm.

You have to pay a close attention to your behavior because there is often a trigger hidden in between your day to day habits. Do you watch television before falling asleep, do you surf the web or read a book? Do you have a coffee drinking ritual with your close friends on daily basis? Try to keep a sleeping diary that will help you understand the patterns in you behavior and also pinpoint the reasons of your condition. In your diary you should note the time when you usually fall asleep and wake up, where do you fall asleep, what you do during the day, what do you eat and drink and also stressful situations that can possibly lead to sleep related problems.

Here are a few tricks that are a precondition for healthy sleep. I know I'm sure that you have heard and read it all before. But it bears repeating again and again until it is second nature. By adopting these habits you could improve your sleeping routine. Worth a try I would say.

   - Make sure your bedroom is quiet, dark and cool. Noise, light and heat can be a reason of an unstable sleep. If you live in a loud neighborhood and do not have a possibility to isolate you from the noise, try using earplugs or a sound machine. Do not smoke in the room where you are sleeping, the scent of cigars is hard to ventilate. Put dark curtains on your windows or use a sleeping mask in order to keep the room dark.

   - Figure out the sleeping schedule to which you are going to stick. In order to maintain your biological clock you should try to fall asleep and wake up same time every day. When is it going to be and also amount of hours slept should suit your needs and organism. You should get back your natural sleeping rhythm, that is why your sleeping schedule should be strict at the beginning, do not avoid falling asleep at the same time even on weekends or when you are tired.

- Avoid naps during the day. Do not take a nap longer than 30 minutes and after 3 pm, because these naps can make it harder for you to fall asleep during the night when you actually need sound and hard sleep.

- Avoid stimulating activities and stressful situations before bedtime. These activities are hard physical exercises, watching TV, using computer or video games, also arguments and hard brainy work. You should try and relax before going to bed. Try out soothing activities as reading something not intellectually challenging or listening to some soft music. Keep the lights low and the room quiet. Try to relax as much as possible using any method you feel most comfortable with.

- Do not use any backlit devices (for example iPad). When going to bed do not read from electronic devices such as iPads. If you use eReaders then purchase one that is not backlit and that requires a use of extra light.

- Avoid or limit caffeine, alcohol and nicotine. Caffeine is not good for your health anyway, but if you cannot avoid drinking caffeine based drinks, and then limit yourself not to use them at least 8 hours before you usually go to sleep. Alcohol is harmful out of many different reasons, but drinking it at the evening can interfere with your sleep. Even though it often makes people sleepy and drowsy it hinders the quality of your sleep. Avoid sleeping before the bedtime and what is a must DO NOT SMOKE IN THE ROOM WHERE YOU ARE GOING TO SLEEP.

If you suffer from insomnia you surely experience anxiety related to your sleeping. You probably can`t stop thinking about your problem and the anxiety level rises when the time for bed comes. You should learn how to associate your bed only with sleep, not the restless nights. And there are some tips that could help.

- Do not use your bed for anything else except sleep and sex. Even though you probably feel comfortable in your bed reading or surfing the web, avoid this habit. You should try to make your brain and body fall asleep when you reach your bed. Avoiding other activities will help your organism to get the signal that it is time for sleeping when you get to your bed.

- Do not force yourself to sleep. When you try to fall asleep and can`t get out of the bed. You should not associate the bed with the awaken state. When you notice you have troubles sleeping get up and do something else in order to feel sleepy again.

- Move bedroom clock out of your view because constant checking of the clock will put you under the pressure. If you need an alarm use it, but place the clock outside of your view in order to relax and stop worrying about the hours you have left for sleeping.

Make a bedtime ritual to help you unwind before sleep.

Read a book or magazine by a soft light
Take a warm bath
Listen to soft music
Do some easy stretches
Wind down with a favorite hobby
Listen to books on tape or podcasts
Make simple preparations for the next day

Herbs that will help you get a natural sleep

You're probably saying HERBS! Are you kidding me? But actually herbs can have tranquil aromas that can be used in capsule form before bed and of course in tea. Many health food stores carry sprays like Lavender that can be lightly sprayed on your sheets and pillow cases. This is my absolute favorite thing to do.

Azahar - This is the petals of citrus aurantium, Amara, or the bitter orange tree species from China. This plant has different benefits for the organism and it is used due to its health advantages. This plant has an antispasmodic effect and sooths the central nervous system, it also improves respiratory problems, it is also known because it lowers the stress. The best way to use the plant is to scent the room where you sleep.

Passiflora - Passion flower - The aerial parts of Passiflora incarnata L effects your organism as a sedative and it also has an antispasmodic effect. The central effect is the depressing of the central nervous system and that is why the plant is used for sleeping disorders, but also anxiety disorders. Stress and anxiety are the most common causes of insomnia and different types of sleeping disorders, so if you have noticed that stress prevents you from sleeping, this plant will help you in coping with insomnia. This plant is available in form of tablets, but also in a form of mother tincture.

Chamomile - Chamomile is known for its soothing effect that helps you calm down and depress your central nervous system. You can try and drink a chamomile tea before the bedtime. Chamomile is also used in form of drops and you should use 30 drops before bedtime.

St. John`s Wort - This plant is known as a natural antidepressant and it is proven that it helps in lowering the anxiety. The herb can be bought in form of tablets and tincture. Due to the fact that Wort is photosensitizing, if you use the herb you should protect your skin from the sun.

Lavender - Lavender is known for its positive influence on different aspects of health and its pleasant scent. If you want to use it in order to improve your sleep the best way is to poor a few drops in your bath before going to sleep. It is also common to use it in a form of tea, but when cooking the plant loses some of its benefits.

Valerian root - Valerian root is famous for its sedative and hypnotic effects. It also improves muscle spasm. Different studies have proved that using of this plant can improve acute insomnia, especially the types of sleeping disorders provoked by somatic manifestations of anxiety. It is advisable to use it in the form of a tincture in combination with other plants according to symptoms.

Kidron - This herb is known for its multiple positive effects. It has an antitumor, antibacterial, antihistamine, anti-inflammatory, antispasmodic but also soothing effect. Due to the multiple benefits this plant can help you in overcoming your insomnia.

Verbena - Plant lowers the level of anxiety and nervous exhaustion. The best way to use it is to put a spoonful of dry fiber in a cup of water and then apply it on the forehead or abdomen.

Self-Massage... Yes!

In order to sleep sound you should relax and calm your thoughts before going to be. Here are 9 steps that will help you achieve this state of mind and further help you get a sound and healthy sleep.

1) Gently massage your hands and fingers; especially take your time massaging your thumbs. You do not have to know any special technique; just use any movement that makes you feel relaxed. Take your time and enjoy, concentrate on the feeling. If you want, you can also use your favorite hand cream or some warm essential oil, perhaps made of herbs that we have suggested as a natural remedy.

2) Rub your palms vigorously for 30 seconds to 1 minute in order to make them warm. Place your hands on your face to cover it whole. Close your eyes lower your shoulders and take 3-5 deep breaths through your nose, exhale through your mouth. This breathing technique will help you relax and the warmth on your face will calm you down.

3) After warming your face, slowly lower your hands and place your fingertips on your temples. Gently press your temples with your fingertips; it is best if you do it with your thumbs. Continue the breathing technique while you are doing this.

4) Slowly move like you are walking your fingers up and down your nose. Remember to continue deep breathing.

5) Lower your hands and rub your index and middle finger under your chin and around your mouth. Meanwhile, open and close your mouth making long aah, ooh, ee and uu sounds.

6) Stroke under your chin and throat with the back of your hands.

7) Move your fingers around your ears; use the same movement like when you moved your fingers up and down your nose. Gently pull and squeeze your earlobes.

8) Place your hand on the forehead and gently alternate stroke up your forehead. Start from the bridge of your nose to your hairline and over your head. Keep your eyes closed and breathe deeply.

9) Return your hands to your lap and relax. You should be in complete peace with yourself and enjoy that feeling that is flowing over you.

You should adopt this routine and do it anytime you have time for it. As for sleeping, you should do this in a quiet, dark and cool place. The best way is to do it before bedtime. You can use some calming music, candles with a calming scent, essential oils or anything that suits your needs. All the advices you read here are the tried out routines, but they should only be the basis for your actions. By combining and experimenting you should find what it is best for you and what works.

Diets... Do They Help You Sleep Better?

What you eat is what you are. Diet is very important when it comes to any disorder, so it is with insomnia. There are some basic things about your diet that you should remember when having troubles sleeping. Melatonin is proved to be useful in treating sleeping disorders, because it is built the same as the sleeping hormone produced by your body naturally that is why you should try and add food rich in melatonin to your everyday diet. *Tart cherries* are rich in this ingredient. Studies had proven that small dosages of melatonin, about 0.3 mg, approximately one cup of tart cherries juice, or 1/8 of a cup of dried tart cherries, help insomniacs get some rest. Sweet cherries contain melatonin, but in smaller amounts.

Oatmeal, whole grain cereals and breads and all types of complex carbohydrates increase production of serotonin, that will help you fall asleep easily. Serotonin slows the brain and nerve activity and spreading a message of well being through your organism. We have mentioned couple of times that the basic precondition for a good sleep is to be calm and free of stress. What is most important is that serotonin, when it gets dark out, turns to melatonin, whose role in a sleeping rhythm has been explained earlier.

If you have noticed that restless legs keep you awake, it is probably due to the lack of iron or some sort of anemia. This is one of the types of insomnia caused by physical reasons that is why you should consult a doctor. He can prescribe you supplements, but our advice is to try with changing the diet in order to solve your health problem. One of the sources of iron is the lead red meat, but you should keep in mind that you should avoid it for dinner; it is most useful if you eat it for lunch. Oatmeal and whole grain cereals are also rich in iron. Another good choice of meat if you suffer from insomnia is turkey. This meat is rich in tryptophan, an amino acid that is used for producing serotonin. In order to make your body produce these substances in bigger amounts try honey with warm milk. A fast digesting carbohydrate like honey, or mashed potatoes for example helps the body to release the insulin, which is crucial in order to tryptophan enters the body.

One additional tip is a bedtime snack. A light bedtime snack can make you feel sleepy. If you are feeling hungry there are small chances that you will fall asleep easily. Take care not to eat too much. The best snack could be something rich in carbohydrates; because it will help to produce serotonin.

How to Eat for Better Sleep

It takes more than ditching unhealthy foods and fun drinks with umbrellas in them. These rules sleep experts swear by:

Don't skimp and splurge.

Missing midday meals may seem like an easy way to lose weight, but doing so can throw off your body's normal sleep pattern. A big meal increases the blood flow to your digestive tract, and makes your muscles work harder. This stimulates your system instead of calming it.

Eat early and often.

Your body uses energy during the sleep process and it needs to be put back. Eat a mix of protein and carbs for. Eating something every few hours helps your body maintain balance.

Just Say NO.

Say no to, cheese plates, and mini meatballs. High-fat, spicy, greasy foods help spark indigestion and that can keep you up long past your bedtime.

Eat carbs for dinner.

Recently a study found some people who ate jasmine rice before bed fell asleep faster or so says the *American Journal of Clinical Nutrition*. Foods high on the glycemic index can help increase the body's production of tryptophan, an amino acid that makes you sleepy.

Don't go to extremes.

Try not to let your calories dip below 1,200, or you might miss out on key nutrients, and this may affect your sleep,

Strike a balance.

A well-rounded diet with foods high in B vitamins, calcium, and zinc could help you rest better.

Don't overdo the salt or coffee.

Most processed foods like deli meats contain lots of sodium, that can interrupt sleep by raising your blood pressure and dehydrating you, Caffeine in coffee, stays in your system for up to 12 hours, so the effects of a p.m. cup of coffee could linger till midnight.

Do go herbal.

Before you go to bed, have a cup of chamomile tea. The plant may act as a mild sedative, calming your body and helping you sleep soundly.

Vitamins and Minerals better sleep

These vitamins and minerals can help you snooze soundly tonight.

B Vitamins

They improve your body's ability to regulate its use of sleep-inducing tryptophan and produce more system-calming serotonin.

These vitamins can be found in things like Chicken breast, lean beef, salmon, bananas, and potatoes, cereals fortified with B3 or B12

Calcium

This is a natural relaxant that has a calming effect on the body's nervous system.

Found In: Low-fat yogurt, milk, cheese, fortified orange juice

Zinc

Deficiency in this mineral has been often been linked to insomnia.

Found in: Oysters, beef, Alaska king crab, fortified cereal

Iron

A lack of this mineral can cause symptoms similar to restless leg syndrome.

Find It In: Oysters, clams, beef tenderloin, dark-meat turkey

Copper

This substance can regulate serotonin.

Found in: Whole grains, beans, nuts, potatoes, dark leafy greens

Bedtime Snacks Less than 200 Calories

You can choose one of these combinations; the fifty-fifty mix of carbohydrates and protein ups sleep-inducing serotonin levels.

- 1/2 cup whole-grain cereal with 1/2 cup nonfat milk
- 6 ounces low-fat yogurt and a sprinkling of berries
- 1 slice whole wheat toast and 1 tablespoon peanut butter
- 3.5 ounces fat-free vanilla pudding and 4 graham crackers
- 1/2 whole wheat pita and 2 tablespoons hummus
- 1 oatmeal raisin cookie and 8 ounces skim milk
- 6 whole-grain crackers and a small handful of walnuts

- A Paleo diet can have an effect on chronic diseases associated with secondary insomnia. Diabetes can be associated with sleep disturbances, and a Paleo diet low in processed starches and sugars is an effective way to manage diabetes. Thyroid problems also respond to Paleo, as do some chronic infections especially autoimmune problems.

- A Paleo diet might help to manage the symptoms of primary insomnia, and help prevent or treat the conditions associated with causing secondary insomnia. Diet alone might not be enough to give you total relief, but it can be a solid first step and a great foundation.

Vegan Diets

Five plant-based foods to help you get a better night's rest.

1. Bananas

Bananas are high in potassium and magnesium, which are natural muscle relaxants. They contain amino acids that help your brain produce the chemical serotonin, which helps you to fall asleep. They contain 110 calories per serving and no fat; bananas are an all-around great bedtime snack. Eat a half a banana an hour or so before bedtime.

2. Cherry juice

Some research has shown that cherry juice may help treat insomnia. Cherries are one of the really rich fruits that may produce melatonin, the hormone that regulates your sleep cycle.

3. Whole Grain Bread

Whole grains are high in fiber which can help keep you full and asleep throughout the night.

4. Seeds

Those people who are deficient in magnesium often suffer from long-term sleep deprivation. Eating seeds like pumpkin, sesame, and flax is a great way to get more magnesium in your diet and thus help you sleep more soundly. Like bananas, pumpkin seeds also contain tryptophan, the serotonin-producing amino acid. Pumpkin seeds also contain high amounts of zinc, which helps the brain convert tryptophan into serotonin

5. Green, leafy veggies

Foods high in folate can help promote sleep, Green leafy vegetables like kale, spinach, and collard greens are high in folate as some experts have suggested aids in better sleep.

Finally Scientific Proof for Beauty Sleep

Beauty sleep is one of those invented phenomena that parents use to make their children get to bed. But now a new study out of Sweden suggests there may be something to it after all.

For the study, 23 participants, all between the ages of 18 to 31, were recruited. They were asked to sit for photographs in the afternoon, between 2 p.m. and 3 p.m. The volunteers were not allowed to consume a mid-afternoon caffeinated beverage to keep them going.

Each photograph was identical — lit the same way, the same distance from the camera, with no makeup and natural hairstyles. The subjects were told to have a relaxed, neutral expression. They weren't allowed to drink alcohol for the 48 hours prior to the experiment. The only difference among the volunteers was that some had had a full night's sleep the night before, while others had been awake for 31 hours straight, after just five hours of sleep the previous night.

The photos were then shown to a group of 65 different people, who, knowing nothing about how tired the people in the photos were, rated their attractiveness. The observers rated the sleep-deprived as less healthy looking, less attractive and, obviously, more tired-looking

Of course, anyone who's ever pulled an all-nighter knows that it's no formula for good looks — the next day, you're saddled with puffy, bloodshot eyes, dark circles and a grey complexion — but now there's a study to prove it.!

Conclusion

I hope this book was able to help you develop habits that will aid you in better, sounder and more restful sleep.

The next step is take action, eat better, shut off electronics earlier, have a cooler darker bedroom and use a combination of any of the many other ideas contained in this book.

To your health and success...

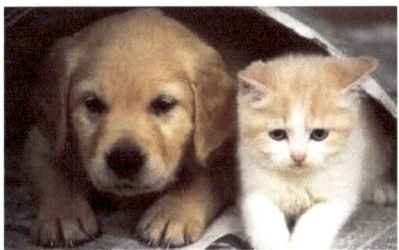

Before you go, I'd like to say thank you for purchasing my book.

I know you could have picked so many other books to read on better sleep.

 But you took a chance on me.

So A Big thanks for downloading this book and reading it all the way to completion.

Now I would like to ask a _small_ favor.

Could you please take a minute or two to leave a review for this book on Amazon?

Click here

The feedback will help me continue to publish more kindle books that will help people to get better results in their lives.

And if you found it helpful in anyway then please let me know :-)

Thank you and good luck!

To your success,

Michele

Preview of My New Book

Listening Skills: Master The Art Of Listening And Communication Skills For A More Confident Life

CHAPTER ONE

Have you ever heard someone repeat the old saying that religious people have been using since someone drifted off while they were speaking? God only gave us one mouth and two ears so that we would listen twice as much. Well, I'm not an overly religious person and I'm not sure that I have the answers to the Cosmos or the greater questions in life, but I do have a response to that. It's pretty much true, in a sense.

If there is one thing that can drive a man or woman insane is the scenario that no one will listen to them. Ever want to communicate something only to have someone completely miss what you're saying? It's enough to make your hands clench into a fist and your blood boil. There's a reason for this.

There are many who believe that the greatest desire of the human being is to be understood and the key to being understood is communication. Communication brings us together, binds us, inspires us, educates us, enlightens us, and relaxes us. It's the way intimacy is built and it's the way validation is given. Without communication, we are entirely isolated in a world that we don't entirely understand and that can be stifling and terrifying to man. But the key to communication is that there are three aspects to it. They are thought, vocalization, and interpretation. One is the art of the mind and how to think of things. The second is the art of the mouth and how to coin those thoughts into a medium by which we can share or test these thoughts. But for us, the focus is the art of the ear, receiving the words of others so that they might inspire our minds or that we might help them.

While we spend copious amounts of time shackled to our minds and often feel the urge to spread our ideas, thoughts, or questions; we are very diligent in neglecting the art of the ear. Our ability to truly listen and understand others is very hard, because it's something we don't always want to utilize and that becomes a problem. If you don't listen to your friends, your coworkers, or your wife; then you're destined for failure in your relationships.

That's why the art of the ear is vital for you to understand if you want to boost your relationships. So here's the rub for you. If you want to energize, invigorate your relationships, then you're going to want to take this book and study it closely because there is one thing that I can promise you. The more you utilize your ears, the more you will inspire and influence those around you to keep coming back. Those who listen more than they talk give off the aura of wisdom, intelligence, and more than that, it isn't a lie. It isn't wrong. Do you understand that? People who listen more than they talk are wise and they are intelligent. Because in the end, you'll understand that there is more to the world that you can learn by listening and the more you learn the smarter you are and the wiser you'll become.

If you want to be a sage person and to experience life without actually having to go through the suffering and the pain of hurts and wrongs; then start listening. People will be inspired by you, they will come to you, and they will invest their lives with you if they know that you're willing to truly listen to them. This is something that you're bound to find out if you just take the time to study the art of the ear.

So whether you want to inspire your coworkers, influence those around you, or find that deeper level of intimacy with your spouse, then take notes, keep an open mind, and start utilizing the things you learn here the moment you put this book down. I guarantee that you'll start seeing the difference immediately in those around you.

CHAPTER TWO
The Ballad of the Man Who Wouldn't Listen

Now we all know someone in their life that wouldn't actually listen to them, but more importantly, we all know someone who has screwed up their life royally by not listening. Sooner or later, there's a person who gets their life completely into the dumps, sucked down in the muck until there's nothing that can really save them all because when it boils down to it, it comes down to not listening.

Click here to read the rest of

Listening skills

Additional Recommended Reading

Sleep Smarter: 21 Proven Tips to Sleep Your Way To a Better Body, Better Health and Bigger Success
by Shawn Stevenson

Thrive by Arianna Huffington

P.S. You'll find many more books like this and others under my name Michele Gilbert.

Don't miss them... here is a short list.

Stop Playing Mind Games: How To Free Yourself Of Controlling And Manipulating Relationships

Instant Charisma: A Quick And Easy Guide To Talk, Impress, And Make Anyone Like You

Chakras: Understanding The 7 Main Chakras For Beginners: The Ultimate Guide To Chakra Mindfulness, Balance and Healing

Practicing Mindfulness: Living in the moment through Meditation: Everyday Habits and Rituals to help you achieve inner peace

Introduction To Palmistry: The Ultimate Palm Reading Guide For Beginners

Emotional Intelligence: How to Succeed By Mastering Your Emotions And Raising Your IQ

Wicca: The Ultimate Beginners Guide For Witches and Warlocks: Learn Wicca Magic

The Introvert's Advantage: The Introverts Guide To Succeeding In An Extrovert World

Adrenal Fatigue: What Is Adrenal Fatigue Syndrome And How To Reset Your Diet And Your Life

Body Language 101: What A Person's Body Language Is Really Telling You...And How You Can Use It To Your Advantage

The Arthritis Pain Cure: How to find Arthritis Pain Relief and live a happy pain free life!

The Headache Pain Cure: How to find Headache Pain Relief and live a happy Pain Free Life!

Stop Panic Attacks and Anxiety Disorders without Drugs Now!: Overcome Panic, Stress and Anxiety and live a happy pain free life!

The Breakup Recovery Guide: Advice for Surviving Heartbreak, Letting Go and Thriving in an exciting new life!

The Friendship Guide to Finding Friends Forever: How to Find, Make and Keep Quality Friendships After your Breakup

The Credit Fix: Leave behind credit card debt and poor credit scores and get your life back!

How To Stop Being Jealous And Insecure: Overcome Insecurity And Relationship Jealousy

The Breakup Recovery Guide: Advice for Surviving Heartbreak, Letting Go and Thriving in an exciting new life!

The Friendship Guide to Finding Friends Forever: How to Find, Make and Keep Quality Friendships After your Breakup

The Credit Fix: Leave behind credit card debt and poor credit scores and get your life back!

How To Stop Being Jealous And Insecure: Overcome Insecurity And Relationship Jealousy

About Michele

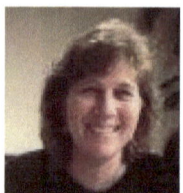

Michele Gilbert was born and raised in Brooklyn, New York. Drawn to literature and writing at a young age, she enrolled at Brooklyn College and majored in English. After graduation Michele did not begin writing immediately, instead she embarked on a career in the finance industry and spent the next thirty years on Wall Street.

Serendipity struck when she least expected it. After ending a long-term relationship, Michele found herself lost and unsure what the future held. She began to read books on grief and loss, looking for answers. Those led her to delve deeper into the Law of Attraction and its power. What resulted was remarkable. Not only had she begun to heal, she had also rekindled her former love of writing and discovered her life's purpose.

The years have taken her through many twists and turns, but she learned valuable lessons along the way. Today she publishes books-mostly self-help and metaphysical in nature-and feels compelled to share her knowledge with those facing similar experiences. Her greatest hope is to inspire others and show them ways to overcome adversity and gracefully accept life's inevitable low points.

Going forward, she plans to incorporate more teachings of self-help, finance and meditation. Regular meditation is very beneficial to her progress as she forges a new life. Morning rituals and positive incantations are other practices Michele embraces; they are very restorative in daily life.

As an avid hiker, Michele and fellow club members often hike the picturesque Jersey Pine Barrens. She is a history buff, voracious reader, baseball fanatic and a foodie. She also proudly supports Trout Unlimited-a national non-profit organization dedicated to conserving, protecting and restoring North America's Coldwater fisheries and their watersheds.

Michele currently resides forty minutes from Atlantic City and the Jersey Shore. She makes her home with a Blue Russian rescue cat named Jersey, though she isn't exactly sure who rescued who.

Michele really enjoys publishing books that can make a difference in people's lives. If you have any suggestions or would like to have a specific topic covered in a future book, please send an email to michelegilbertbooks@gmail.com and we will get back to you.

Thanks for reading!

www.ingramcontent.com/pod-product-compliance
Lightning Source LLC
Chambersburg PA
CBHW050918290526
45792CB00002B/797